Emerging from the Storm

Harriet Knock

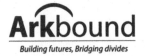

Building futures, Bridging divides

Emerging from the Storm
by Harriet Knock

ISBN: 9781912092581

First published in 2020
by Arkbound Foundation (Publishers)

Arkbound is a social enterprise that aims to promote social inclusion, community development and artistic talent. It sponsors publications by disadvantaged authors and covers issues that engage wider social concerns. Arkbound fully embraces sustainability and environmental protection. It endeavours to use material that is renewable, recyclable or sourced from sustainable forest.

Arkbound
Rogart Street Campus
4 Rogart Street
Glasgow G40 2AA

www.arkbound.com

Emerging from the Storm

I would also like to dedicate this to my two perfect sons Freddie & Edward.

They are my anchors and keep me grounded.

RE-IGNITION

My dear, although right now you may feel weak,

Let me assure you that life won't always look so bleak,

You see, you are far from obsolete,

You just need something more to feel complete,

I ask you to look deep within your being,

Find the things that bring you happiness and give your
life meaning,

Endeavour to do more of what makes you smile,

I am sure life will seem much brighter in just a short while,

Spend more time surrounded by those that you treasure,

Maybe it will bring your life more pleasure,

You see, things right now may look foggy and dark,

But I promise, if you don't give up, you can reignite the spark,

You will feel happy and once again you will smile,

For now you must simply take the first step of the mile,

The journey to happiness is never fast,

But as soon as you get there long may it last.

Gone be the liar,

Over be the fight,

I know you begin to tire,

I beg you don't lose sight,

When the battle is over,

When the war is won,

I hope you feel the closure,

I hope the pain is gone,

I hope the joy spreads like wildfire,

I hope your heart burns bright,

May your eyes beam with desire,

May you radiate the light,

The truth is we all deserve to live,

We don't need to destruct our self,

We too deserve the love that to
others we freely give,

We can win against mental health.

ANXIETY

I suffer from anxiety,

But I am still me...

Doing my best to fight it and
trying to be happy,

I suffer from anxiety and it
affects me every day,

I can't explain this feeling, it
presents itself in so many ways,

I suffer from anxiety but I am
strong enough to fight,

I will not let it ruin my life, I'll
face it with all my might.

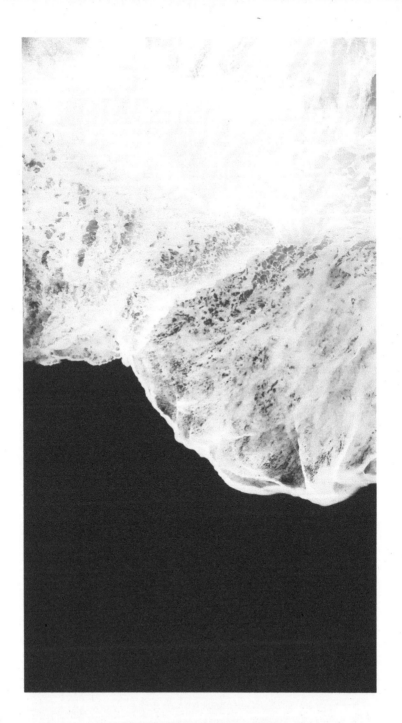

FAKE A SMILE

They tell you just to smile,

Like it will fix everything,

I've been trying for a while,

Faking it's so tiring.

It's strange because others just
don't seem to see,

That it's just a mask and deep
inside I'm really not happy,

If they tell you to fake it,
please don't feel like you must,

If you're feeling that rubbish just
speak to someone you trust,

Faking a smile gets you nowhere
if you're dying inside,

They say fake it til you make it,
but I didn't make it, they lied.

Sat in a dark room crying because all you want
is to be free,

Consumed by depression and mental health,
how strange to think that used to be me,

Even the people smiling that now seem so
carefree,

There's more to us all and our past than the eye
can possibly see,

I promise you, you can recover and there's
more to life than you think can be,

Strength comes in numbers and support so
instead of 'you' fighting it's 'we',

I used to be the one suffering in silence alone
curled up small in my bed,

I thought I was the only one fighting such awful
feelings inside my head,

Now I'm strong enough to discuss it and my aim
is to help give someone hope and see the light,

There's more to life than this feeling, you can
turn it around if you fight,

I promise you, you can be happy, although this seems
hard to believe,

With support of your friends and family, you'll be
surprised at just what you can achieve,

When I look back to my past and the place I was in it
feels like a distant memory,

I didn't think life was worth living, I just wasn't happy
being me,

Now I am through that dark tunnel I smile when I
look back to where I was then,

Because although it was awful and traumatic, I'm
confident I'll never be there again,

I now have so many reasons to smile and so many
blessings to count,

I have had my fair share of dark and difficult moments
but grown stronger by an incredible amount,

I just want to help someone know,

That you really are not alone,

No matter how bad things get, just be assured it's not the end of the road,

The future for you is bright, I'd never have guessed what life had in store,

I now have a beautiful family who I really do adore,
I now have a genuine smile,

Trust me recovery is so worth while,

I now have so many things to be grateful about,

And I hope to help someone else by speaking out,

Each day you fight your strength and bravery is admired,

But please get the help you deserve and require,

It doesn't mean that you're failing or make you look weak,

But your life could be saved if you just open up and speak.

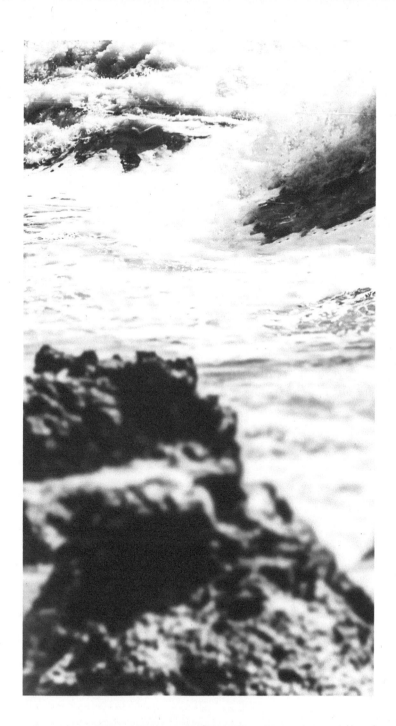

Mental health problems are so very real,

It's important to address our emotions
and talk about how we feel,

You could save your own life if you just
open your mouth and shout,

Even if you whisper, or cry, or scream,
it's just better to get it out.

Locking up those feelings,

Is more damaging than you know,

Take it from someone who's been there,

I didn't know how to let anything go,

Inside my mind was a battlefield,

I was tormenting myself all the time,

I wish I could've dealt with things differently,

Instead of punishing myself like a crime.

Anxiety has got me again, its gripping
me by the throat,

As much as its trying to drown me,
I'm determined to stay afloat,

Anxiety has got me again, its' hand
covering my mouth and nose,

I'm struggling to breathe now, I wonder
if it shows,

Anxiety has got me again, it feels like
I am suffocating slowly,

Yet from the outside I still seem fine to
all of those who know me,

Anxiety has got me again, I've won once
and I'll win once more,

But oh it is so tiring, constantly fighting
your own mind is such a chore,

Anxiety has got me again, why do I never
feel enough?

I know that I am strong... But why is life
so tough?

Anxiety has got me again, no words really
can explain,

How something in your head can cause
this amount of pain,

Anxiety has got me again but together
we can pull through,

So take my hand, be brave and smile,
we will win, we always do.

Breathe in, breathe out,

Don't scream, don't shout,

Breathe fast, breathe slow,

Don't stress, just let it go,

Sometimes things are beyond our control,

Remember not to panic, just keep your feet on the ground,

In life, experiences can take their toll,

We must learn from the situation and turn it around.

Anxiety can knock me down and
wipe me off my feet,

Anxiety can weaken me but never
will I be beat,

Anxiety can make my stomach sick
and make me physically shake,

Anxiety keeps me up at night,
worrying myself awake,

Anxiety is awful and really hard to
understand,

So if you know someone is struggling
please lend a helping hand,

When you're sat there night or day,
or lying in your bed,

With a thousand worries and doubts
all swirling round your head,

Please know it's very normal and
you're really not alone,

There's so many of us struggling and
it's ok for you to moan!

If you need someone to talk to, please
never be scared to speak out,

If you want someone to talk to, you
can message me, just shout,

Anxiety is not a weakness, anxiety will
not beat us.

If you're feeling anxious just know you're
never on your own,

No matter what time of day, there's always
someone at the end of the phone,

If you're feeling anxious, stressed and maybe
worried too,

Just look at how far you've come and how
many people believe in you,

If you're feeling anxious just remember to
breathe deep and slow,

Hopefully soon this feeling will pass and the
panic attack will go,

If you're feeling anxious just remember that it
won't last,

Every bad day and moment will soon become a
part of the past,

If you think you can't do this or you really feel
you can't cope,

Remember your record for getting through bad times is 100% so don't lose hope,

If you're feeling anxious just know that you are not to blame,

Sometimes the way our mind treats us feels like we're losing some kind of game,

If you're feeling anxious just remember that you're loved by lots,

These people will support you whether they get what you're going through or not,

If you're feeling anxious, just know that you're stronger than you think,

Sit down and take just five minutes to calm yourself with a hot drink,

If you're feeling anxious, in that moment it can be hard to know what to do,

So use your phone as distraction if needs be, someone will be there to speak to you.

We need to talk about the problem that is mental health,

Something that affects not just those living in poverty but also those living in wealth,

Something that affects girls, women, boys and men,

You don't know if it will impact you, you won't know why or when,

Mental health has no target audience so no one is protected,

If your mind get poorly it's important it's not neglected,

If you injured your body or broke your arm,

You'd go to the doctor and show them the harm,

So why if you're broken deep inside,

Do people assume its best to hide?

Please talk about the problem and tell someone what's wrong,

Before the damage can no longer be undone,

Mental health is NOT taboo,

It has happened to me, it could happen to you!

It's something so common so why are we hushed,

People must learn to speak before their limits are pushed,

Too many lives are taken by illness of the brain,

So many people suffer without anyone else knowing they're in pain,

Lets end the stigma and help each other to talk,

If mental health tries to drag you down, tell it where to walk,

We can all beat it with adequate support.

There is a whirlpool of emotions,

Whirring round my brain,

There is a whirlpool of emotions,

Driving me insane,

There is a whirlpool of emotions,

I am drowning in the pain,

There is a whirlpool of emotions,

Trying to ruin me again.

I often wish, that I could turn if all off,

I often wonder, what silence would feel like,

With no worries, no doubts and no criticism
in my mind,

I wonder how I would enjoy to relax and what
it would feel like to unwind,

You see my mind does keep me busy, it keeps
me on my toes,

Always panicking and overthinking, inventing
the unknown,

Situations that will probably never happen but
they still consume my day,

If only I could turn it off, if only I knew the way.

Sometimes people need to take a pill,

Sometimes it helps to control the raging
feelings that eat us up,

Is it really any different to taking a painkiller
for a broken limb?

When we need something to numb the pain
that's crippling us from within,

I think pill shaming needs to end, it should be
seen in a different light,

Just because mental illness isn't visible,
shouldn't invalidate the fight,

Take that pill if it helps you, don't worry what
others may say,

Sometimes we just need a helping hand to
make it through another day.

I am a worrier,

Though I am a warrior,

Many a time have I lied,

When someone's asked how I'm doing inside,

You see I am a worrier,

But as I fight it still,

It also makes me a warrior,

For battling on as I will.

The pitch black night is rolling in,

Suffocating my soul,

All sense of direction is now lost,

All peace and calm is gone,

I can't explain how depression feels,

Because everything seems numb,

I often wonder why I deserve this,

Is it something that can be undone?

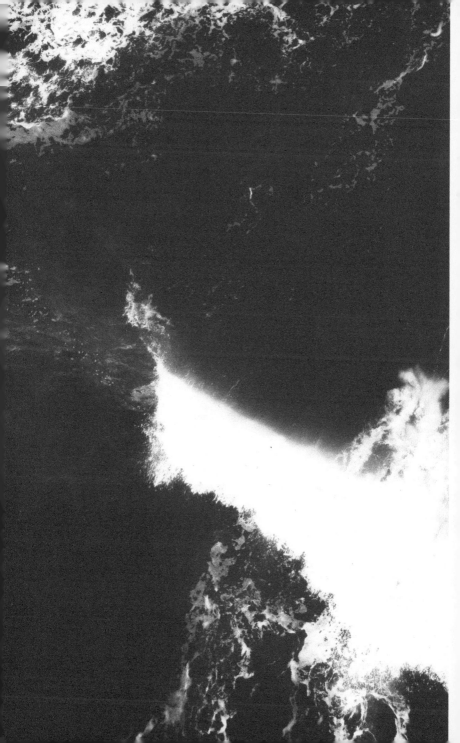

Lying beneath the sky,

Awaiting the beautiful sunrise,

Each day is a brand new chance to shine and glow,

Each day brings new lessons to make us change and grow,

You see just like the bright, warm sun,

We too will rise again, once each day is done.

You need not wait for a new year to change
your resolutions,

Each new day, hour or minute, can bring the
chance to start again,

A new beginning can be had with every single
breath,

Align yourself with a new path to reach your
current goal,

Or reassign yourself a new sight to aim for,

One thing is certain, you must keep moving
forwards always,

One small step in the right direction will get
you miles further than any step back.

It was just a bad day today, I didn't feel
I would make it through,

But here I am, making it, and tomorrow
is fresh and new,

Another day, another start,

A fresh chance, a forgiving heart,

Each bad day will soon be over, so close
the book each night,

And when the sun does rise, welcome it
with open arms and make things right.

Once upon a time I thought my life was over,

But it's never over yet!

There's always a reason to fight,

There's always a purpose don't forget.

Suffering from anxiety is like
struggling to swim,

When you're stuck out in a rip
tide, and the storm is rolling in,

Suffering with anxiety is like
floating when you can't fly,

Wondering how you got in this
mess and asking yourself why,

Suffering from anxiety is like not
wanting to leave your home,

It's the fear of what is out there,
what could happen if you roam.

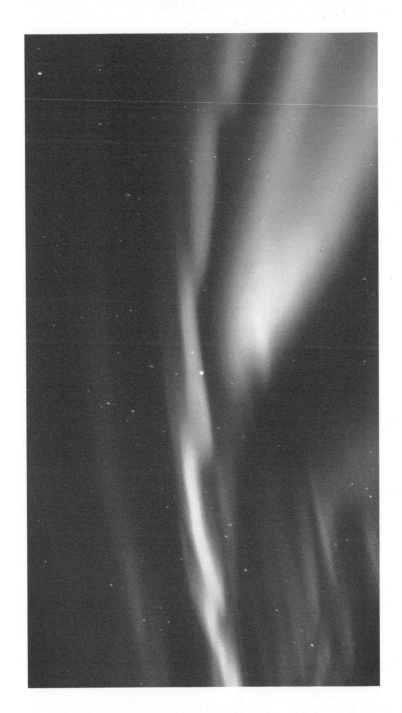

PRESSURE

There is a constant pressure in my mind,

Am I not enough? Am I too much? Will
I be on time?

Asking myself these things constantly,
unable to unwind,

I feel this age should bring happiness,
I'm basically in my prime,

But I feel I'm wasting so much of my life,
by fighting the demons constantly,

I wish I could just live freely, instead I feel
controlled by me,

It's such a weird sensation when your mind
is fighting you,

We're meant to live in unison and just live
as one, not as rivals in two.

BRIGHT

In time, things can and will get better,

One day the sun will rise and it will be
different to before,

A different light will dance through the
curtains and cast across your floor,

A different smell will linger and your
spirits will slowly rise,

A different feeling will rush over you
and take you by surprise,

Things can and will get better, I've seen
it with my eyes,

You see there is such thing as hope and
things will start to look bright,

One day you'll think back to these
words and surely I'll be right.

Once upon a day, not so long ago,

I thought my life was over, little did I know,

Literally things change over night,

I felt the spark return, I felt compelled to fight,

Just like that I turned my life around,

Within myself, finally, happiness I found.

I am my own worst enemy,

I am kind to others but not to me,

I need to learn to love myself,

To benefit my mental health.

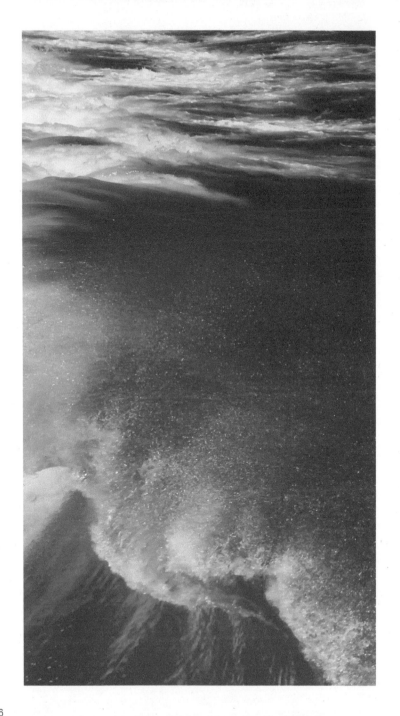

APPEARANCE

Don't count your stretch marks
or dwell on your saggy skin,

Don't worry about your weight,
just love yourself from within,

Stop panicking about fitting
back in to your jeans,

Learn to live with your new
body and love it by all means,

Recovering from an eating
disorder puts us through
so much,

So please be gentle and kind to
your body with every little touch,

Don't fret about your appearance
or how you may have changed,

Look at yourself as magnificent,
amazing and slightly rearranged.

Right then in that moment,

I realised this is so much bigger than me,

So many others are suffering in silence,

Feeling lost and very unhappy,

Unsure whether to speak up, who to talk to, or what to do,

So keep plodding along, its the only way to pull through,

One day your life could change, just like it did with mine,

I used to have to fake it but now I mean it when I say I'm fine,

I'm now genuinely happy with my smile in its place,

When once upon a time only tears ran down my face,

The key is never give up on life when you don't know what could be,

It cannot rain forever,

One day it will be sunny.

It is extremely hard not to panic when that feeling
weighs down in your chest,

When you realise you're really struggling even though
you're trying your best,

It's important to remember that this is not your fault
or choice,

Mental health problems can affect any of us but please
do find your voice,

Going to the doctor, or seeking professional advise,

Will help you to get better, even though admitting
how you feel isn't nice,

It can be hard to talk about, it can be difficult to say,

Just how low you're feeling when you're having a
bad day,

But with support in place, you will be able to heal,

The things that you're experiencing are very real,

You deserve to recover, you deserve to have a hand,

I know you will get over this, I'm living proof you can.

RELAPSE

A relapse is when it doesn't go to plan,

When you feel like you can't and it all comes crashing down,

If a relapse happens, you need to remember you can,

A relapse is not a nice thing to go through,

When it feels like all you have achieved will suddenly undo,

Please remember recovery isn't linear for you,

A relapse does not mean that you cannot start again,

You can pick up from where you left off,

Instead of having to re-begin,

A relapse is not the end of the lane,

Recovering is a long, slow process, but worth it,

It's time to keep on moving, away from all this pain,

A relapse happens when we're pushed to the test,

So maybe take a breather,

It's sometimes vital just to rest,

A relapse is just an obstacle or a blip,

Keep on jumping hurdles,

Shake yourself off and get a grip

A relapse is a normal part of recovery for some,

Do not panic, don't give up,

Remember where you're going and how far you've come.

LOST

I'm lost, I'm lost,

Why can't you see me?

Between the green and shaded trees,

I'm sat there begging on my knees,

Why me? Why me?

Why do I feel this bad?

I'm just so tired of feeling this sad,

I feel so empty, I feel so down,

I cannot smile or even frown,

My mind is empty, my face is blank,

I'm lost, I'm lost,

Please find me.

A friendly voice called through the trees,

Shouting come out and show yourself please,

They sounded gentle, they sounded kind,

A very different voice to the one in my mind,

I stood up tall and faced my fears,

I approached them, drowning in salty tears,

I cannot do this, I'm not enough,

I'm strong but this life is far too tough,

They took my hand and guided me,

And showed me what it's like to be free,

They told me their names are hope and faith, they
made friends with me,

And said that to meet with them again I must believe,

So from the woods I walked, still broken,

But with new strength after words were spoken,

I feel a fate is waiting for me somewhere,

Now I need to keep going until I get there

I ask that you open your eyes today,

And look at the world in a different way,

Fear not of the dangers, don't be afraid of
what could go wrong,

Live for the risks, life is not all that long,

We must be brave and take a stance,

We must give this life our best chance,

Time is short and the years are fast,

We must spend it making memories to last.

Ana, Ana, my friend Ana,

She told me food is bad,

I never thought I'd beat her but
now I have I'm glad,

Ana, ana, my friend ana,

She told me I'm too fat,

I thought I was and starved myself
to get the perfect thigh gap,

Ana, Ana, my friend Ana,

Was not a friend at all,

She told me it was better to be skin and
bones,

I was so weak I could fall,

Ana, Ana, my friend Ana,

Tried to ruin my life,

She told me it was ok to feel weak
as long as I was light,

Now I realise how evil she is and that all
those things weren't right,

Ana, Ana, my friend Ana,

This one is for you,

I'm now the heaviest and healthiest I've
ever been, and that's no thanks to you.

ANOREXIA

The number on the scales,

Consumed my every thought,

The idea of gaining a pound,

Would make me feel distraught,

My weight was all that concerned me,

Skinny was all I really wanted to be,

I wanted to see how light I could get,

It was like some kind of twisted bet,

Between Anorexia and Me.

FAT

Fat fat fat,

How about that?

I hated my body and living in
my own skin,

It's awful feeling insecure and
hating yourself from within,

Fat fat fat,

I am not that,

There is so much more to us
than our shape and our size,

If your mind is not being nice
to you, don't listen to it's lies.

Some days are sent to test us and
take us to our knees,

These days are to strengthen us,

Life is tough but we are tougher,

Some days are rough but we've
faced rougher,

The world is hard but we are strong,

We've known it's a test all along,

So keep on facing it every day,

Despite mental health problems,
we're here to stay.

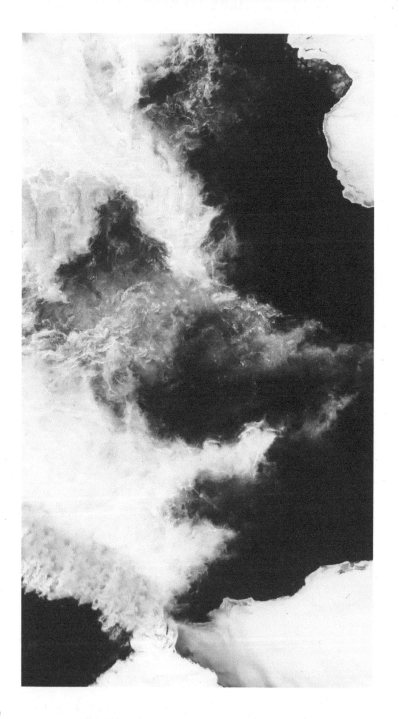

A MOTHER'S SUPPORT

My Mother told me it broke her heart,

To hear of how much I was torn apart,

See at the time I hid it well,

But now, standing brave, my story I'll tell,

It took a lot of time to feel ok,

It won't get better in just a day,

I hate to think of what my Mother must
have felt,

To see how much I was struggling with
all these problems I'd been dealt,

But if it wasn't for her support I don't
think I would still be here,

I'm so thankful that she held me despite
each falling tear,

A Mothers support does have no price,
something I will never be able to repay,

But if it wasn't for my Mother holding me up,
I doubt I'd be standing here today.

I wake up every morning with a smile on my face,

Knowing that in this huge, vast world I've finally found my place,

I walk around each morning and in my step is a spring,

Because I am ever so grateful, since this new life did begin.

Getting better took so much time,

Even now I have dark moments,

But it is so different now,

A bad day is just a bad day,

Not a storm like it once was,

I know that I can swim through the waves,

When before I could not,

It's not about trying to stop the rain,

It's about learning to dance through it,

Until the rain is no more and you are free of pain.

If I can do it,

You can do it,

If you can do it,

We can do it,

If we can do it,

Then there is no stopping us,

Mental health will not defeat us.

This world is so big and scary, it's hard to visualise,

That within this whole universe we all share the same skies,

So don't judge the person struggling,

Don't judge those hiding away,

Don't judge the person crying,

You don't know what they have been through today,

Sometimes we are fighting a silent battle inside,

And no one else would even know as it's so easy to hide.

Be kind to one another,

Be loving and gentle in all you do,

But remember as well as giving it freely to everyone else,

You need your own love too.

Self care is not just taking a bath,

Sometimes it's as simple as getting out of bed,

That task can be the hardest when you're fighting
your own head,

Self care is not just taking a walk or meeting
up with a friend,

It's surviving and getting through another day
when you've been wishing life could end,

Self care is not just getting a make over or
painting your nails,

It's keeping it together to brush your teeth when
you feel like flying off the rails,

Self care is not just reading a book or listening to
your favourite song,

Self care is reassuring yourself that you're doing
ok and not doing everything wrong,

Self care is so important and even small acts will
help, from showering, to brushing your hair, or
eating something good,

I'm proud of you for trying, even when you didn't
think you could.

Feeling sick,

Feeling numb,

Feeling stupid,

Feeling dumb,

Know it's silly,

Can't make it stop,

Feeling so anxious,

Another tear drops,

Sweaty palms and trembling,

Everything's overwhelming,

To everyone else it's a simple thing,

I can't stop overthinking.

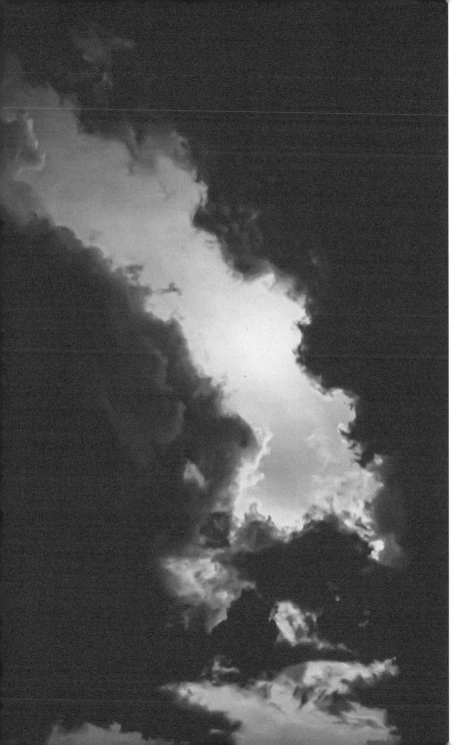

Bleeding gums,

Tangled hair,

Aching from head to toe,

Panic attacks,

Heart palpitations,

No one else would know,

Sweaty hands,

Tired eyes,

Nightmares every night,

No proper meals,

Feeling drained,

Everyone thinks you're alright,

Nails are brittle,

Skin is dry,

Eyes are full of tears,

You just seem fine,

You've nailed it now,

You've been faking it for years.

SIMPLE THINGS

The thing about anxiety is no one else can see,

Just how overwhelming and scary these simple
tasks are to me,

I find it hard to make a phone call,

I find it hard to leave my home,

I don't know what I'm scared of,

Is it the unknown?

I feel a little silly,

I wish I could be free,

Of this awful mental health problem,

That keeps controlling me.

The truth is I sometimes can't face
stepping out of my front door,

If I'm having a bad day I stay in my
safe place when I feel raw,

The truth is even when we're healed
experiences can still be there,

It's important to recognise your own
triggers so you can be aware.

Don't feel bad if you need to rest,

When life has put you to the test,

When your limits are pushed and you're feeling weary,

Remember that things won't always be seen clearly,

Sometimes life can leave you feeling blurry,

When everything happens in such a hurry,

It's hard to keep your head screwed on strong,

When a voice is constantly telling you, you are wrong,

So take it easy and please do rest,

Don't beat yourself up if you're doing your best.

On ourselves we are too harsh,

We are not kind or forgiving,

So speak to yourself as you would speak to a friend,

And start to love the life you're living,

Life is too short to beat yourself up over and over again,

You need to let the sunshine in and let go of the rain.

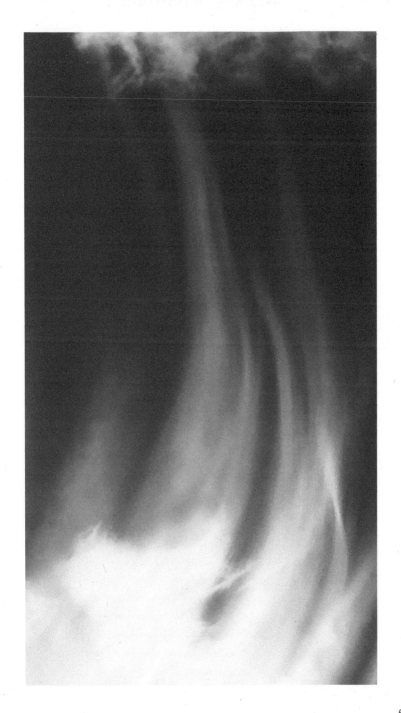

The only person in control of you is you,

It's in your power to change your life if
you really want to,

It's hard to start with and it takes time
but trust me it's a worthy tale,

Just get back up and keep on trying,
regardless of how many times you fail.

IT'LL SOON BE OVER

Bad days come but bad days go,

It'll be over much sooner than you know,

So ride it out and hold on tight,

Soon everything will be alright.

Hard times shape us,

Hard times break us,

Hard times prepare us,

Hard time create us.

BLISS

Never have I felt anything like this,

So settled and content, floating in bliss,

Living in a paradise,

Where everything is nice,

Gone are all the worries of the past,

I wish I'd known they wouldn't last,

That one day they'd be but memories,

And the bad times would no longer effect me,

Now I just feel so free,

A new start, a new happy.

ONE DAY

What if I told you one day it would all change,

If life was like a puzzle piece you could simply rearrange,

What if I told you it doesn't have to be like this,

There will be a time that's settled and not so hit and miss,

The future is uncertain but you can shape it too,

I just can't wait to see what time will bring to you.

I now feel so much more sane,

Than when I was fighting my own brain,

I now feel so much more stable,

When before I just thought I was unable,

I now feel so fresh and revived,

Everything I've been through and still I have survived!

THE MASK

I may look strong,

I may look brave,

You are wrong,

It's the illusion I gave,

Behind this mask is the real me,

To others I fake it and look happy,

It's easy to lie and it's easy to hide,

The emotions that we are actually feeling inside,

Don't be quick to judge,

Let go of the grudge,

We never know what others feel,

Behind the fake shared highlight reel.

Don't let go,

Recovery is slow,

Don't let go,

You will survive and you will grow,

Don't let go,

Just go with the flow,

Don't let go,

Tell your demons 'no',

Don't let go,

You will stand another blow,

Don't let go,

One day you'll say I told you so,

Don't let go,

You won't forever feel this low,

Don't let go,

You are stronger than you know,

Don't let go.

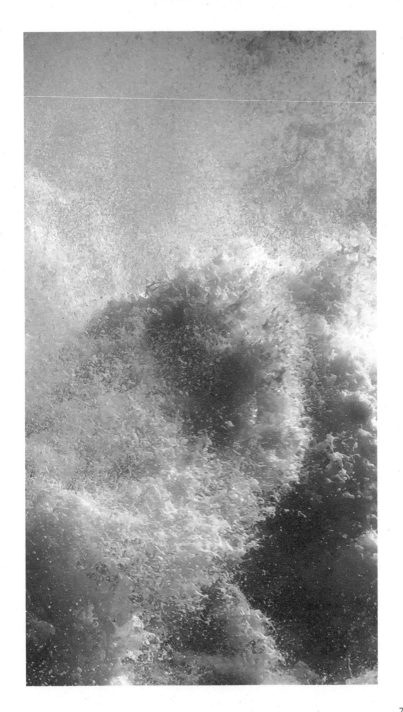

I will hold you through each dark, cold night

I will take your hand and be your guiding light

I will reassure you that soon things will be alright

I will stand in your corner and urge you to fight.

Just like a mother, I'll stay by your side,

Just like a mother, I'll be there as your guide,

Just like a mother, I'll support you on this ride,

Just like a mother, from me you cannot hide,

Just like a mother, I'll know if you have lied,

Just like a mother, I'll wipe the tears you've cried,

Just like a mother, I'm proud that you have tried,

Just like a mother, I'll still be filled with pride.

WAVES

The ocean is created

from many smaller rivers

A tide is created

from little ripples like shivers

The ripples travel through my body

like a tidal wave

The stormy sea is crashing down

but I know I will be saved.

The worries in my mind are weighing down so heavy,

I'm walking, unguided, on trembling feet unsteady,

In all honesty I don't know if I'm quite ready to face,

This overwhelming journey where I hope to find my place,

The first step is the hardest, it's the biggest of them all,

But I must keep moving forward and get back up if I fall,

The universe is spinning and never will it end,

I need to find my happiness so that my soul will mend.

I have anxiety,

Anxiety does not have me,

I know I will get through this,

I know I can be free,

Goodbye anxiety, you cannot
dull my shine,

I'm taking this life back now,
as afterall it's mine.

AS BLACK AS THE NIGHT

The darkness rushed over me as black as the night,

It muffled my senses and blurred my sight,

The worry sank heavy like a ship out at sea,

The feeling of my heart, like an anchor, drowning me.

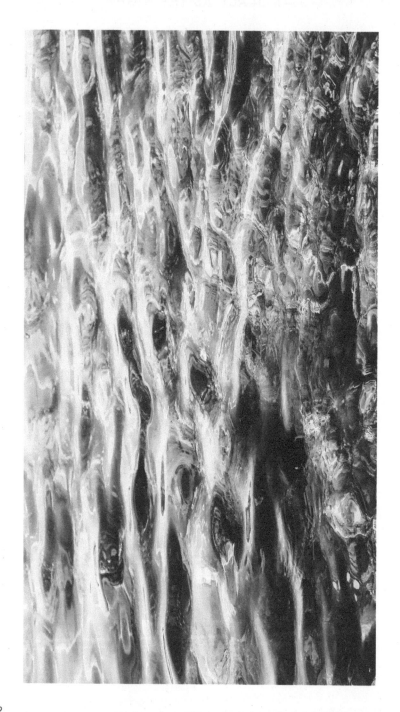

TRAIN TRACKS

The ringing sounded through my mind,

A vision of those I'd be leaving behind,

One step forward, one step back,

Hesitating whether to step on the track,

Then something clicked, I turned and ran,

I didn't think I could fight this, then realised I can,

Hold onto your nearest, live to see their smile,

Remember you'll only feel this way for a short while,

Feelings are temporary, ending your life is not,

Don't even think about it, give happiness another shot.

Depression, depression, what can I say,

It affected my life each and every day,

I felt so empty, I felt so numb,

I wondered if it could ever be undone,

I now realise that it wasn't my fault or choice,

I had to learn to fight myself and find my inner voice,

I now have gained strength and courage too,

Going through these awful times have changed my
point of view.

No one in their right mind
can understand a lost soul,

Unless you've been in the wrong mind
and had to guide yourself back whole.

It's hard to comprehend,

Wanting your life to end,

When you've never experienced the dark,

If you've never fallen apart,

It's a feeling from within,

To describe... I can't even begin.

SELF HARM

Self harm was an escape,

Self harm was a way to cope,

Self harm was an alternative,

To a noose made out of rope,

Self harm stopped the feelings,

Of wanting to end my life,

Self harm gave me a way to escape,

When the emotions got too rife.

Although it may cause alarm,

The truth is I used to rely on self harm,

It's true when they say you bleed to know you're alive,

At the time it was the thing helping me to survive,

The thing no-one tells you is it's like an addiction,

But they all think you're crazy and that's your conviction.

SCARS

Scars are something that we have all got,

Whether they are visible, whether they are not,

Scars are formed when we have been through pain,

When we win a battle, thats when a scar is gained.

HOLD ON

Back in the past, I wanted to end my life,

I never thought I'd be a mother or one day become a wife,

Life can change so quickly so please don't give up yet,

If you just hold in there, you'll be happy soon I bet.

REMINDER

Run the bath, Make the cuppa,

Read the book, Watch the movie,

Listen to the song, Look after your being,

Not just your surroundings,

Look after the mothership,

Not just the offspring,

You cannot keep holding up others,

When you don't have the strength to stay up yourself,

Take time for you, Take time for the little things,

It makes all the difference,

If you give more to yourself, You have more to give
to others.

Sometimes when I wake I don't want to
get up out of bed,

Sometimes I don't want to brush my teeth
and I don't want to fight my head,

The thought of facing another day can fill
my mind with dread,

Sometimes at my lowest I have wondered
if I'm better off dead,

Sometimes it's the little things that really
seem so hard,

I wish I could live another life by swapping
my hand of cards,

Sometimes I can't face anything and don't
want to brush my hair,

Sometimes there's dirty washing and dishes
everywhere and I really couldn't care,

Sometimes I just feel empty and like I'm
slowly suffocating,

Sometimes I wonder if I really matter, so
I just keep isolating,

Sometimes I feel so lonely even though I
know I'm not alone,

Sometimes it feels impossible to even
answer the phone,

You see mental health is real and so many
of us struggle,

Fighting your mind and trying to be strong,
really is a juggle,

For those who do not suffer it must be
hard to comprehend,

How someone can wake up some days
just wanting life to end,

For those who also suffer I'm sorry no
words can make it right,

But please don't ever lose hope and never
give up the fight,

For us this is our story and we should not
be ashamed,

Our mental health problems are not our fault
and for how we feel we won't be blamed.

I CAN

I turned my hopes into dreams,

I turned my wishes into plans,

I worked hard and instead of 'I can't',

I told myself I CAN.

Please don't judge if my home is sometimes messy,

I'd really rather live like that than constantly be stressy,

Please don't judge me if there is laundry everywhere,

Or if I'm still in my pyjamas and I haven't brushed my hair,

Please don't judge me because you really have no clue,

Just how much responsibility I have and how many things there are to do,

I may have overcome the worst of my struggles,

But now I simply have so many things to juggle!

It's only now that I have walked along
this dreary road,

That I understand just what it's like
to carry such a heavy load,

To feel so burdened and have to
wander without sense of direction,

To fight so blindly without support
 or the safety of protection,

Now I know how tough I am,
I really put up a fight,

And although I'm finally recovered
now, believe me it took all my might.

THE PITS OF DEPRESSION

In the pits of depression,
you don't hear them shout or cry,

In the pits of depression,
you don't hear the truth or lies,

In the pits of depression,
all you feel is numb,

In the pits of depression,
all you love is gone.

Please hold on, don't lose hope,

Step off the chair, untie the rope,

I know it can seem easier to leave,

But think of those left behind to grieve,

I promise you life won't always be this way,

You just need to hang on and take it day by day,

One day your life can change and it will,

Just hold on in there, don't let depression kill.

I've been at the bottom,
I'm now at the top,

As soon as I started smiling again,
it's been impossible to stop,

I've cried in the shower,
I've cried in the rain,

But now I'm smiling happy,
without an inch of pain,

They say that time's a healer,
just wait and you will see,

One day you'll be much happier
and come out on top like me.

STAND UP TO YOUR DEMONS

It's hard to be positive when you
can't see the light,

It's hard to win the battle when
you've no energy to fight,

When you get through this you'll
feel really glad,

You won't always be unhappy,
 you won't feel forever sad,

You need to hold your fists up high
and tell your demons they won't win,

You need to win the war,
just use the power you have within.

It is easy to surrender and admit defeat,

Being defeated won't get you anywhere,

It is easy to give up and say you're beat,

Instead of lying there, get up and fight for those that care.

I am happier now than I have ever been before,

All the darkness of the past kept behind a closed door,

I am more whole now, than I have ever even knew could be,

They say a tiger keeps its stripes but I am definitely a new me.

Mental health problems are seriously scary,

It is hard when your mind makes you overthink and feel wary,

It is draining when you are fighting yourself inside,

Because you are the only person from which you cannot hide,

You need to slowly teach yourself love,

You need to change the way you speak to yourself from your mind above.

BROKEN

Bruises, cuts,

They all think I'm nuts,

Crying, screaming,

Nightmares when I should be dreaming,

Feeling empty, feeling numb,

Not drinking a drop, not eating a crumb,

Destroying myself from inside out,

Dying so silently but wanting to shout,

No-one would listen, no-one would care,

Although someone is, I feel no-one is there.

I look out of the window, the sun is rising
slowly ahead,

It makes me smile softly, I am glad I got
out of bed,

Today is a good day, though that won't
always be the case,

I know I will get through it all, I've been
in a much worse place,

You see we must be grateful for the beauty
the whole world holds,

For all the memories we will make, for all
the stories which will be left untold,

We must live for the unknown moments,
we must live to see what's in store,

You see what we can behold with our eyes
is nothing, to life there is so much more.

BLOSSOM

Happiness radiates through me like the blood flowing
through my veins,

I never thought I would feel this alive and this inspired,

I feel like I was buried, but really I was planted,

As now I have grown and blossomed into my true self,

I truly believe each experience is sent to shape us,

I now realise the value of time, time I spent feeling hurt,

It was teaching me to grow, keep an open mind and push
on through the dirt.

Always pursue your dreams,

Even if life feels ripped at the seams,

Always set your goals higher,

Aim to reach for what you desire.

FREE

Place your feet on the ground and slowly breathe,

Stand and exhale as you count from one to three,

Pick your chin up and know that you're free,

Whatever is burdening you, stand tall and let it go,

You are in control of your life, just take it slow.

THE ROSE

As the last petal on the rose does droop,

I sympathise as I too know what it is like to wilt,

Without love or nurture,

Without food or water,

All of a sudden, it doesn't look so beautiful anymore,

All that was is gone,

Bare,

No petals, no colour, no beauty,

But unlike the rose,

My petals grew back,

One by one,

Until I was more magnificent than ever.

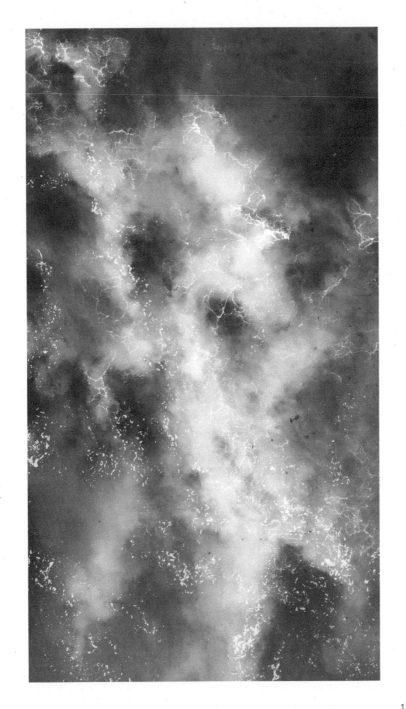

ABOUT THE AUTHOR

Harriet Knock is currently a stay at home Mum to her two toddlers, grasping the opportunity to follow her dream!

Finally with enough time to dedicate to her passion of writing, she is able to share the story of her battle through mental health problems, and the victory of recovery, through emotive poetry.

It is a dream come true to have her first book published, something she never imagined would become a reality.

If we share our stories we can inspire others, Harriet is passionate about raising mental health awareness and hopes this book will be able to provide hope and comfort, while shining a light on the topics often left in the dark.

Together we can break the stigma around mental health problems, raise awareness and encourage people to fight, seek support and begin the road to recovery.

ND - #0430 - 270225 - C0 - 197/132/7 - PB - 9781912092581 - Matt Lamination